Why write about surveys?

Developing surveys is not celebrated work and suffers a poor reputation for a multitude of reasons. Most notably, the tools required for effective survey design are based in cognitive science, statistics, research methodology, human and social behavior--as well as clinical expertise. Unfortunately the complexity is often under-appreciated. Not just by those of us that design and write them but even by organizations requesting data.

Many of the great advancements that have been made in digital environments have not been adopted by survey methodology in healthcare or medical education. The abuse of survey analytics and burdensome question fatigue and lack of relevance makes it easy to see why there is a lack of interest—even disdain—for survey design.

I am writing a book to change that perception. Survey development and implementation remains the best way to gather knowledge from a sample that hopefully will provide information about a larger population. It's the difference between fishing with a net or a harpoon. The large net will have a lot of smaller collateral information to distract and distort the primary purpose. Think like the fisherman highly skilled with a harpoon. Stay on point.

Take heart, survey designers. The journey will be long, but our cause is just.

Much of what I learn happens during conversations, personal interviews, and observations. I want to share that here. Research methodology is a dynamic field of inquiry. Understanding what makes our findings relevant and informative requires an appreciation for behavioral economics and cognitive behavior.

Why start here? If you are interested in collecting your own data whether it is from electronic health records, medical education conferences, or population health at the patient or community level--how you ask the question is as important as what you are asking. The insights included here are the "most bang for your buck".

There will be more. Once you are able to collect data as objectively as possible—the sky is the limit. We can tackle data visualization, improving numeracy in medicine, preventing overdiagnosis, health policy and health economics, and many more topics.

If you can stop making the mistakes highlighted here you will immediately benefit. It isn't about spending more money or needing to hire a research methodologist or survey expert--it is about learning a few simple skills--and unlearning a few low-value habits that are ruining your insights, research, and outcomes.

I have used all of the top survey analytic tools at one point or another. As long as there is a no-cost option or free trial during the steep learning curve, I am a fan. Qualtrics has been my preferred analytics tool because it integrates well with my data visualization tool--Tableau. But don't fear the monkey.

Survey Monkey is a decent point of entry as well. I do find that self-designers often fall victim to fancy widgets in "pro" version upgrades from free trial software. Be cautious. How you collect the data influences how you are able to interpret your findings.

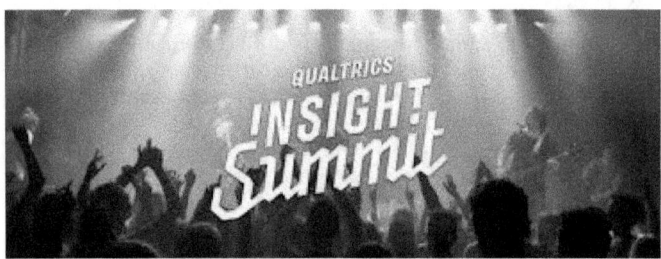

I traveled to Qualtrics Insight Summit conference in Salt Lake City, Utah hoping to discover new innovative engagement strategies in survey design and insight analytics. The survey instrument is the most common data collection tool that I rely on to field behavioral gaps and measure baseline competence. I learned a lot. How to design better surveys, increase response rates, convince decision makers, and tell the stories the data tell us.

A few fresh best practices can help you gain actionable insights without too steep of a learning curve. Data strategies fall flat if you are struggling to find value or meaning from the data you are collecting. The worst feeling as a data analyst is having loads of data rendered meaningless by vague and misleading questions, biased answer choices, and poor planning. Think of the old adage—pay now or pay later.

Writer Better Surveys. Period.

Copyright 2016 Bonny P McClain
Published by Data & Donuts

Acknowledgements

I would like to thank all of the terrible surveys that I may have written earlier in my career, the spurious data generated by surveys others have written, and a certain tenacity that made me believe we can do better.

I would also like to thank big data for being such a red-hot mess. We greedily grab at the possibility of your revelations to guide or force our insights. But most of all, I would like to thank the outliers--the little data points existing at the long tail. Thank you for allowing me to tell your story. We can all do better by driving real insights within our research, stories, or organizations.

Thank you to my own little data universe—my family and little "n of 4". We strive to do better every day. Continue the journey. You never know the difference you might be making.

Creating your visualization

When I begin to design a survey I typically create the report or slide presentation first. The research going into a topic can set the foundation for the type of data, audience, and research design needed to gather meaningful information.

- What data will you need?
- Think about the variables you would like in your ideal data set
- How will you visualize your data?
- What questions will you need to ask?
- Do you know how to ask them in a way that will yield accurate data?
- Do you know how to clean or restructure your data?
- What are you comparing?

You can pull your report together and move through the list above. What questions are you interested in exploring? The first step will be identifying the right type of data. What data sources are available? I am looking at the right level of granularity? Population level? Patient level?

Once we narrow the focus we can search for sources of the right kind of data. There are quite a few databases available online for free or a minimal fee. What types of variables are you interested in measuring? Costs? Payment for services? Geography? Pre-planning how you want to slice the data can save significant time in finding the right information. I often use the United States Health Information Knowledgebase (USHIK). You would be surprised how many of your peers don't even know it exists.

"The United States Health Information Knowledgebase (USHIK) is an on-line, publicly accessible registry and repository of healthcare-related metadata, specifications, and standards. USHIK is funded and directed by the Agency for Healthcare Research and Quality (AHRQ) with management support and engagement from numerous public and private partners."

This is perfect world survey design. We don't need a funder. We just need a research question clearly defined with appropriately selected comparisons.

W.E. Deming is considered the father of quality control. An engineer and statistician tasked with helping Japan recover economically after World War II, he may know a thing or two about performance measures and evaluation strategies. He made an important distinction between enumerative and analytic studies. Prior to reading his seminal papers, I basically lumped all my surveys into one bucket. Shame on me.

Enumerative and analytic studies differ based on action. You need to determine the type of statistical study because the specific action you engage depends on the part of the population accessible to your analysis.

For example, an **enumerative survey** basically calculates a frequency. *How many?* You are limited to the population you queried. You can chop up the normal curve of the data you collect from the population you sampled. An analytic survey evaluates the process or system that produced the outcomes. **Analytic surveys** are asking "*Why?*"

What drove the differences in frequencies detected in the enumerative survey? Our questions require consideration of what comes next—how to improve behavior or practice sometime in the future. Looking for differences between groups. You can continue to gather data from new distributions as you strive to reduce the variability in the data—between the current measured value and the optimal behavior or outcome.

How accurate are surveys?

I will provide a list of resources at the end of the book to help guide those of you wanting a deeper dive into the research methodology of survey design. My intention for the majority, if not the entire book, is to provide a conversational less scholarly overview of what I have learned over the years from conferences, experts in the field, writing really awful surveys, learning to write better surveys, analyzing terrible surveys (from large companies that should know better), and the literature.

When I say "less scholarly" I am referring to limited journeys down research methodology historical precedence. The research has been done for you. Here are the outcomes for your consideration.

Linchiat Chang and Jon A. Krosnick

National Surveys Via Rdd Telephone Interviewing Versus the Internet: Comparing Sample Representativeness and Response Quality

Public Opin Q (2009) 73 (4): 641-678 first published online December 1, 2009 doi:10.1093/poq/nfp075

It is easy to point a finger at errors in survey design. Selecting the wrong populations, not adjusting for non-responders, errors in measurement but what do we know about accuracy? How accurate are they? The answer is, pretty accurate. A meta-analysis conducted by Chang and Krosnick used the following methods to assess survey accuracy:

• Match each respondent's self-report with objective individual records of the same phenomena
• Match one-time aggregate survey percentages and means with available benchmarks from non-survey data
• Correlate individuals' self-reports on surveys with secondary objective data
• Correlate trends over time in self-reports with trends in objective benchmarks

These findings are a welcome relief. Surveys are designed, implemented, and analyzed based on the fact that they are relatively accurate approximations of reality.
The study provided objective evidence across a wide variety of metrics using a variety of methods –

   "*Comparing each respondent's self-report with objective individual records of same phenomena; correlating aggregate distributions of respondents' reports with distributions of same phenomena derived from secondary data not based on self-reports; comparing one-time aggregate survey estimates with available benchmarks; and comparing trends over time between longitudinal aggregate survey estimates with available benchmarks.*"

So now that we know that the "juice" is worth the squeeze, how do we get started?

Better question design--improving reliability and validity

Survey research methodology isn't sexy. I get it. We want to write our questions, cross our fingers, and send the survey out into the ethos. Hopefully after a few days we have enough engagement to say something thoughtful about our specific query. Trust me on one thing. It isn't that easy.

"The principle of satisficing can also be applied to events such as filling in questionnaires. Respondents often choose satisfactory answers rather than searching for an optimum answer. Satisficing of this kind can dramatically distort the traditional statistical methods of market research."—The Economist

There are behaviors that distort our findings. Take satisficing for example—it is real and if we don't attempt to minimize the behavior in our survey design—all the hard work is for nothing. We discuss satisficing in detail later on...stay with me.

I am not delusional. In my experience, the resources allocated to front-end survey design are often nonexistent or relegated to a senior level manager or writer /editor. I am certainly not an expert in research methodology but I do have a theoretical grasp of the latest literature and experience developing robust outcome analytics and survey assessments.

There are wide gaps between what is happening in daily practice and what high quality survey instruments look like. Most of us, unfortunately, are not taught to necessarily appreciate how bias, poor question design, poor answer choices, and undefined measures can render the data and potential summations meaningless. The survey design is envisioned as a list of questions—nothing more nothing less.

My goal here is to make us all a little better. Even though I spend a big chunk of my day working on analytics and designing surveys – you don't have to do anything drastic. Stop doing the bad bits and replace old habits with new insights. The latest blockbuster drug is the patient survey. You know the buzz words—patient reported outcomes, shared decision making, physician insights...It should be easy to tackle the design in-house or without consideration of cognitive biases or awareness of poor question design.

But first consider your goal. You are requesting information from a respondent. Each question has to be reviewed for potential alternative interpretations. Next, consider any socially desirable influence that may distort the response. If you are fielding Likert scales, data shows a skew toward the extremes in questions of agreement or assertions. And finally, **does the context of the question influence the meaning?** Let's look at some of these practices in detail…

What types of questions are best?

Historically I avoided open questions like the plague. Before easy access to optical character recognition (OCR) software, the task of evaluating the responses was manual and slow—if you were lucky. There are two scenarios when you should lean toward "open" questions. If the universe of possible responses is vast—for example, in a qualitative survey—or if you are tempted to include an "Other" option on your survey consider writing a few "open" text questions.

Expecting a respondent to effectively engage using a text box is going to lead to disappointment. People tend to be attracted to pre-defined responses so better to keep it open. I do need to remind you of the extra time needed to code "open" text. Let me include another plug for data visualization. You can generate bubble diagrams to help sort common keywords quickly for hypothesis generation.

Ranking questions vs. rating scales

I am a recovering Likert addict. What can I say? Rating seemed so easy. You can jam quite a few of these types of questions into a survey without too much resistance. Here is the problem. What if you wanted to rate a list of treatment options for a particular clinical condition? In reality, all of the behaviors could receive the same rating. You need relative importance or preference—you need a ranking question.

This may be a new question type for you to consider. You may be surprised to learn that your survey platform includes ranking as an option. Voila! If so, there are a few options. A full ranking of objects allows absolute comparisons. This type of data is highly reliable. It might look like a list of treatment options under consideration for a presented case study.

Partial ranking might work better. Too long of a list will force your respondents to the extremes. Trust me on this one. You can always ask for a respondents "top 3" or "bottom 3" and help them along their way. Minimal ranking is probably the least informative but you can easily determine the extreme for the most important or least important.

Ranking questions are easiest in self-administration questionnaires because respondents are able to view all alternatives. But please be aware--ranking is a difficult cognitive task and can be time consuming for the respondent. Also the data analysis is more complicated.

Let's get back to discussing rating questions. The omnipresent Likert scale uses rating questions to measure opinions and assertions on a variety of topics. Do you want to know how much someone learned? Use a Likert (pronounced Lick-ert).

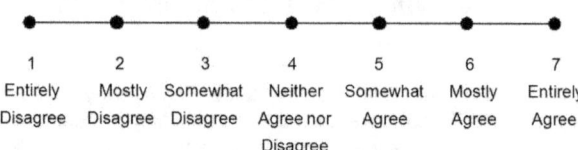

1	2	3	4	5	6	7
Entirely Disagree	Mostly Disagree	Somewhat Disagree	Neither Agree nor Disagree	Somewhat Agree	Mostly Agree	Entirely Agree

A common "no--no" rampant in survey design arises when coding numeric values inconsistently. The Likert scale should include a value for each statement—much better than just coding the extremes and allowing respondents to make a vague decision regarding intensity.

The proper Likert scale is also directional—the highest value should correlate with the best outcomes. The problem is not readily corrected if the wrong direction is coded. If you have unknowingly flipped the scale you cant be certain that respondents went along with you for the ride. They may have assumed convention thinking the right edge of the scale was for better outcomes or perhaps indeed followed your reverse scale. You will never know. It is better to standardize the scale once and for all and be consistent.

Likert scales are easier for respondents to complete, easier to analyze but they also lead to lower data quality. Responses toward the end of the survey will be less reliable. Your data will also be "noisier".

During survey data analyses I have always had a preference for 7-point scales. When you are writing survey questions you need to be able to differentiate between meaningful levels of a construct. Come to find out there is a bit of science behind when to select a 5-point scale or a 7-point scale.

It depends on the scale you are using. Are you using a *bipolar* construct? Think of these as a good to bad scale with a neutral midpoint like "disagree and agree" scales, for example. Bipolar constructs are best with a 7-point scale with a neutral midpoint.

An example of a *unipolar* construct is a 0 to positive scale. A 5-point scale works fine—always with a neutral midpoint. Always label the scale points. Why? The objective is for all respondents to interpret the meaning of a scale the same. A scale like the Net Promoter Score for example, is ambiguous with out labels for each point. Respondents will be disproportionately attracted to the points that are labeled. Label them all.

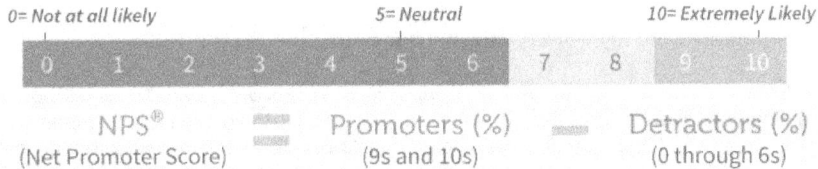

Writing survey questions—go time

How should I word my word/phrase my questions?

My first bit of advice about writing survey questions sounds like my advice on writing learning objectives. Always think about the number of verbs in a question or learning objective as a red flag. You don't want to be double-barreled. I recently adopted an easy check to find double barrels. Do a search for "AND" in your survey. If you find it—you likely need to delete everything that follows the "and" or split it into two separate questions.

The overarching goal in question writing is "meaning uniformity". To the best of your ability, each question should mean the same thing to all respondents. You can come closer to the goal if you write succinctly. Be careful of words with variable meanings, too many syllables, or industry jargon.

It is easy to assume that our audience will know the abbreviations or jargon from our industry but what happens if they assign even slightly different meanings to the words? It could nudge responses along a scale in either direction.

Word selection guide:
- Words a clear meaning
- Fewer syllables
- Simple sentences avoiding homonyms (fare/fair) and heteronyms (lead/lead)
- Avoid negations (this means those awful "**which of the following "isn't**"…)

Does the order of questions matter?

You probably know the answer to this one. It is likely you have taken your share of surveys along the way. I have written more than I can count and frankly, the hardest habit for me to break was opening with demographic questions.

When you appreciate the cognitive demand of a well-written survey it becomes clear why we should park those least demanding questions to the end. Save the early real estate for important topics.

If you are including "open ended" questions consider asking them in the beginning of the survey.

Always structure questions from general to specific. Once you prime the respondents' brain, group similar topics together. Questions that may tax long-term memory are easier to retrieve cognitively if you have ordered questions appropriately.

Also don't forget we need to think of data in aggregate. When possible, randomly vary question order across respondents (even randomizing within sections can help). Full disclosure I never took advantage of this underutilized methodology until recently. We do know that preceding questions impact responses to questions that follow. To help mitigate any potential bias in how questions are ordered, be certain to use randomization strategies.

A perfect segue for discussions of the pre-survey. Much of the cautionary biases and survey "breaks" (respondents stop responding) can be identified with a pre-survey. You should always send you survey out for review by trusted colleagues, experts in the field, or even friends. A lot can be learned from a few cognitive interviews. Ask your pre-survey respondents about specific responses. What was confusing? What was difficult? What was easy? Pay special attention to broken skip logic, typos, leading questions, and potentially confusing syntax.

I have a small group of colleagues that are happy to field my survey before it is ready for prime time. Why? Hopefully they see the "win--win" proposition. A brief insight into methodology and an ability to ask questions--more often than not, will improve the final instrument. From time to time, you will find out a question can be interpreted different ways. Catching a last minute typo or esoteric word choice is worth its weight in gold.

I see continuing medical education (CME) surveys all the time biased on the answer choices provided. I reviewed several from a leading medical education company that made egregious errors. Failure to screen mental health patients for suicide ideation in critical case studies, avoiding a competitor's drug (standard of care) in the answer options even though it was a first tier drug, and a host of other non-evidence based algorithms. When you take the time to circulate a pre-survey, you can be confident in the underlying framework.

Advanced—writing good questions

It is easier to keep the steps to survey design in mind once you understand the cognitive response process experienced when taking surveys and how they influence data quality.

The respondent has to **understand** the intent of the question, **search** memory for relevant information, **integrate** the information into summary judgments and finally **translate** the judgment into response alternatives.

How can we help respondents to optimize all 4 steps? First, there are a few cognitive short cuts you want to minimize. Our brains are nothing if not efficient. The short-cuts are necessary but we need to be aware where they may be happening—and unintended.

You many not have heard the term satisficing. I used a quote in the first section describing a cognitive short cut experienced when tasks are difficult or the respondent ability is low. Perhaps the respondent has a biased memory **search**. This is a type of weak satisficing. Respondents that skip memory, search, and integration and look for plausible options are more problematic.

Causes of satisficing

Task difficulty (interpretation—too many words complicate retrieval--multiple dimensions), and challenging response selections can all trigger cognitive shortcuts.

Respondent ability is something we can't necessarily control (cognitive skills, experience thinking about topic, pre-consolidated judgments)

Respondent motivation
How motivated is the respondent to complete the survey? Do they have a need for focused cognition? What is their degree of accountability? How about the personal importance of topic, belief about survey importance, or number of prior questions?

How can you recognize satisficing behavior?

Order of response can affect answers
- Visual presentation = primacy (the first reasonable response seen)
- Randomize categorical responses

Agreeing with assertions

Acquiescence bias—we want to say yes.

- Agreeing with assertions
- Agree-disagree (LIKERT)—use different language
- True/False
- Yes/No

Generally avoid any form of these response scales. Use construct specific questions.

Straight-lining or non-differentiation

Do you agree or disagree with the following statements? We called these clinical assertions when I first created outcomes surveys. Avoid grid or matrix questions like these! Mix up response scales! Remember the goal is to minimize generating low quality data.

Including I don't know (IDK) question responses. Avoid these. Not the same as selecting middle alternative/neutral—could just be a tired or unmotivated respondent. Research has shown that respondents provide consistent and accurate responses when IDK removed.

Take home message?

Task difficulty—make questions easier, minimize distractions, and keep the duration short. Also consider moving the more cognitively demanding questions to the beginning of the survey.

Respondent motivation--leverage survey importance, keep duration short, and you can always use incentives and encouragement to increase engagement.

Not another survey…sigh

I write surveys for healthcare stakeholders. This is pretty vague I know but in the era of big data—everyone is assessing and appreciating the value of engagement. Patients, caregivers, healthcare providers, policy makers, health economists, data analysts, we all have a collective opinion and unique insight profile deemed valuable somewhere within the bigger ecosystem.

Tell your potential respondents why you value their input. I can't tell you how many clinicians hesitated to participate when they thought they were providing grist for the pharmaceutical industry mill. But once they see value for their patients or business needs—they are committed. I am also a big advocate of sharing survey findings. You can provide trends or individualized feedback—I leave that up to you.

The most popular (and easiest recruited) surveys I have written were based on retractable barriers for physicians at a crossroad at a clinical decision point (treatment resistant patient populations) or in need of tailored information around a specific business need (EHR functionality and data access).

Does size matter?

How many responses do you really need? True a large sample will yield more accurate findings but unless your budget is large there will need to be certain compromises.

I am going to share a bit of simple numeracy around basic statistics principles.

Before you can calculate a sample size, you need to identify the target population:

1. Population Size — How many total people fit your demographic? Are you looking for patients that fit a certain criteria or diagnosis? You can approximate numbers but it is always better to base it on available data.

2. Margin of Error (Confidence Interval) —The confidence interval determines how much higher or lower than the population mean you are willing to let your sample mean fall. A margin of error of +/- 5% is saying the value might be 5 points higher or lower than what is reported.

3. Confidence Level — How confident are you that the actual mean falls within your confidence interval? The most common confidence interval is the 95% confident level.

4. Standard of Deviation — How much variance do you expect in your responses? I select .5 typically to ensure that a sample will be large enough.

Now you can **calculate our needed sample size.**

Your confidence level corresponds to a Z-score. This is a constant value needed for this equation. Here are the z-scores for the most common confidence levels:

• 90% – Z Score = 1.645 • 95% – Z Score = 1.96 • 99% – Z Score = 2.326

You can find a Z-score table online if you are using different confidence levels.

Plug your Z-score, Standard of Deviation, and confidence interval into this equation:

Necessary Sample Size = (Z-score)2 * StdDev*(1-StdDev) / (margin of error)2

Here is how the math works assuming you chose a 95% confidence level, ".5" standard deviation, and margin of error (confidence interval) of +/- 5%.

((1.96)2 x .5(.5)) / (.05)2 (3.8416 x .25) / .0025 .9604 / .0025

= 384.16

385 respondents are needed

If the sample size is too large you can decrease the confidence level or increase the margin of error – this will increase the chance for error in your sampling, but it can greatly decrease the number of responses you need.

###

Resources

SURVEY RESEARCH
Annual Review of Psychology Vol. 50: 537-567 (Volume publication date February 1999)
DOI: 10.1146/annurev.psych.50.1.537

The Psychology of Survey Response Tourangeau, Rips, and Rasinski (2000) **ISBN:** 9780521576291

The Science of Asking Questions Annual Review of Sociology Vol. 29: 65-88 (Volume publication date August 2003) DOI: 10.1146/annurev.soc.29.110702.110112

Thinking About Answers: The Application of Cognitive Processes to Survey Methodology 1st Edition, Sudman and Bradburn (1996)

Question and Questionnaire Design, krosnick and Presser (Handbook of Survey Research 2010)--
http://courses.ischool.berkeley.edu/i271b/f12/readings/2010HandbookSurveyResearch.pdf

Answering Questions: A comparison of survey satisficing and mindlessness Vannette and Krosnick (the wiley Blackwell handbook of mindfulness, 2014)

About the Author

Bonny P McClain is the founder of Data & Donuts, a well-respected blog written at the crossroads of health economics, health policy, and clinical medicine and research. In 2015, Bonny was invited to the White House to write about the White House Conference on Aging. She continues to report and provide analyses from panel discussions at the National Press Club, Brookings Institution, and scientific conferences such as AAAS, 76th Scientific Sessions American Diabetes Association, Qualtrics Insight Summit, and Tableau Annual Data Visualization conferences.

Bonny has written several books about medical writing and improving numeracy in medicine. When she's not busy traveling for her consulting business you can probably find her out running on the trails, perusing a local art museum, or traveling to the beach with her family. Read Bonny's Amazon profile here http://www.amazon.com/Bonny-P-McClain/e/B00J0M10OY

Other books by this author

Please visit your favorite ebook and print retailer to discover other books by Bonny P McClain:

- 5 Sources for the Right Healthcare Data: Bigger isn't Always Better
- The Learning Objective: Identifying Appropriate Metrics for Improving Medical Education
- Medical Writing for Smart People
- Improving Numeracy in Medicine
- Continuing Medical Education: What to do when good outcomes go bad.

Connect with Bonny

I really appreciate you reading my book! Here are my social media coordinates:

Friend me on Facebook: https://www.facebook.com/dataanddonuts
Follow me on Twitter: https://twitter.com/graphemeconsult
Subscribe to my blog: http://www.dataanddonuts.org
Subscribe to my other blog: http://www.alzheimersdiseasethebrand.com
Connect on LinkedIn: https://www.linkedin.com/in/bonnypmcclain